Physical Pain Herbal Medicine

The 10 Best Solutions to Relieve Back, Neck, and Shoulder Pain

Table of Contents

Introduction

Congratulations on downloading *Physical Pain Herbal Medicine* and thank you for doing so.

Herbal medicine, which is sometimes called herbalism or botanical medicine, involves using plants, or parts of them, to treat illnesses or injuries. This also includes using botanicals or herbs to help a person's overall health and wellness. Traditional medicine practitioners, herbal medicine practitioners, herbalists, and naturopathic, homeopathic, and Ayurvedic healers all use herbal remedies.

Ginkgo biloba is one of the oldest herbs in history. According to fossil records, Ginkgo has been on the earth since, at least, the Paleozoic period. One of the earliest known medical documents was recorded by the Egyptians around 1500 BC, known as *Papyrus Ebers*. This 20-meter long scroll held 700 plant-based remedies.

Shennong Bencaojing, the first recorded herbal study, was written by the Chinese Emperor Shen Nong around 2000 BC. He was known for his multitude of innovations like dietary revolution, seed preservation, and he had tasted hundreds of herbs. His writings contain information and descriptions for 300 plants.

The monks, during the Middle Ages, grew medicinal herbs. The Native Americans gave the colonist herbs and plants like Black Cohosh, which is still used to relieve pain and menopause symptoms 'till this day.

The extracts, flowers, roots, bark, stems, leaves, and seeds of plants have been used in herbal medicine for more than a millennia. These types of treatments have been given in capsules and pills, in liquid forms, as topical applications, in tinctures and teas, and raw. At first, the plants were all consumed raw or mixed with hot water as a tea or soup. In later years, people started drying and crushing the plants for other uses. The plants were discovered in the wild, and they often based their uses on superstitious or visual cues. People would often use plants to treat body ailments because it looked like that body part or because they commonly grew in a certain area. Science helped people to refine the use of herbal remedies. Herbs and various plants are the precursors to a number of modern medicines.

Today there are many modern and Western medical practitioners that turn to herbal remedies for common and uncommon disorders. The lower cost and safer use are very attractive to medical professionals. There are also some physicians who use herbs to help offset the side effects of regular pharmaceuticals.

There isn't an exact date as to when humans started to use herbs for medicinal purposes. We do know that the first written information about herbal medicine dates back to around 2800 BC in China. Since then, the popularity of herbs for pain relief has gained and fallen out of favor several times in the medical field. The following timeline will show you some of the major points in the history of herbal medicine:

- 2800 BC – The first written information regarding herbal medicine.

- 400 BC – The Greeks started to use herbal medicine. Hippocrates stressed out how important overall happiness, exercise, and diet are as the foundation of wellness.

- 50 AD – The Roman Empire started to share herbal medicine throughout the Empire, and with this started the commerce of cultivating herbs.

- 200 AD – The first appearance of a classification system that paired common illnesses with their remedy. This was created by Galen, an herbal practitioner.

- 800 AD – Monks became the rulers of the herbal field with their gardens in infirmaries and monasteries that cured the injured and sick.

- 1100 AD – The new center of medicinal influence was the Arab world. Physician Avicenna wrote the *Canon of Medicine*, which mentioned herbal medicine.

- 1200 AD – The Black Death started the spread throughout Europe, and herbal medicines were used along with the "modern" methods like mercury, arsenic, purging, and bleeding with similar or better, results.

- 1500 AD – Parliament and Henry VII promoted and supported herbalists and herbal medicine, mainly because of the number of untrained apothecaries that gave substandard care.

- 1600 AD – The poor were treated with herbs, while extracts of animals, plants, mineral, and the "drugs" were given to the rich.

- 1700 AD – Preacher Charles Wesley gave herbal medicine another high-profile endorsement. He was an advocate of herbal treatments, sensible eating, and good hygiene for healthy living.

- 1800 AD – Herbal treatments took a back seat from pharmaceuticals. As the drugs side effects started to be documented, herbal remedies gained popularity. The National Association of Medical Herbalists was created, and then later changed its name to the National Institute of Medical Herbalists.

- 1900 AD – During WWI there was a lack of drugs available, and this increased the use of herbal medicines. When the war ended, penicillin was discovered, and pharmaceutical production increased. Practitioners of herbal medicine had their rights to dispense medication taken away and then reinstated. People started to become concerned about the dangerous side effects and environmental impact of pharmaceutical drugs during the '50s.

- 2000 AD – The EU started to regulate and test herbal medicines, like the regulations in pharmaceuticals.

For nearly 4000 years herbal medicines have been documented. This type of medicine has survived real world testing and thousands of years of human use. There are some medicines that are not used anymore because of their toxicity, while others have been combined or modified with additional herbs to help offset side effects. Herbs have undergone changes in terms of how they are used.

Herbal medicine is still popular today. In some ways, it has even gained new momentum. More and more people have started to seek out alternative treatments. As physicians look for new treatments for the most common illnesses, they are starting to look back at herbal medicines.

Typically, today, herbs are cultivated for medicinal purposes. Very few herbs are harvested in the wild, except for those that are located in higher elevations or rainforests.

Elderly people tend to metabolize medications differently and typically take more medications. This means that they need to exercise caution when they try new herbal supplements.

Pain Relief

There isn't a single herb, vitamin, or mineral that offers the same significant level of pain relief that heavy-duty prescription drugs provide. But, natural herbs for pain relief don't come with the side effects of prescription drugs. They are also more cost-effective and don't come with the same risk of chemical dependency.

Certain herbs not only alleviate pain but also address the underlying causes of it and supports and heals the nervous system. There are over 100 herbs for pain relief, and not all of them work the same. Herbal remedies are meant to work alongside with regular pain treatment.

Over 40% of Americans, according to Johns Hopkins University, use alternative medicinal therapies to help control pain when prescription medications aren't working.

Herbal treatments provide individuals who don't have access to pain clinics access to pain relief. According to researchers from the University of Michigan Health System, the most frequent users of alternative pain management are older individuals.

Herbal remedies tend to be less expensive than conventional treatments. There are also a few side effects, although that doesn't mean there aren't any reactions. Depending on the condition or medication that a person is undergoing, they can have a reaction to herbal remedies. This is why it is important to speak to your health care provider first and do plenty of research.

Before we dive into the book, a word of advice, make sure that you talk to your doctor before you start trying any of these alternative pain relief methods. While they are all natural, there is a chance you could be allergic to them, or they could interact with any prescriptions you are taking. I have tried to add in as much information on possible problems, but there could be more than I am unaware of.

There are plenty of books on this subject on the market, thanks again for choosing this one! Every effort was made to ensure it is full of as much useful information as possible, please enjoy!

Capsaicin

A big part of the cuisine in India, Central America, and Asia are chili peppers. In the United States, you can go to any store that sells sauces and find a variety of hot sauces oftentimes with the words "fire," "inferno," or "insanity" on the label.

People love chili peppers because of this heat, and it's also the biggest reason why it has so many medicinal properties, particularly pain relief. The capsaicin found in chili pepper is what gives it its heat. Capsaicin is a compound that the chili pepper produces to protect the pepper from fungal attack. Capsaicin is odorless and colorless, but when consumed, it makes your brain believe that there is heat wherever it comes in contact with your body.

Interestingly, though, birds aren't affected by capsaicin. This makes it possible for them to spread the seeds around so that the plant can survive. Virtually all mammals are affected by capsaicin, although, it's believed that humans are the only mammals who willingly choose to eat them.

How Peppers Tricks the Brain

The nervous system has TRPV1 receptors, which are heat-receptor proteins. These are located in the cells of your digestive system and skin. The receptors are inactive unless a person is exposed to temperatures over 107.6 degrees Fahrenheit.

Once this happens, you will experience pain and heat, which is telling you that you need to move away from whatever is causing this heat. When a person eats a chili pepper, the capsaicin in it will bind to and activate TRPV1. This means that though there isn't any real danger, your body believes that it's being exposed to excessive amounts of heat.

The *New York Times* further explains this:

"... in mammals it stimulates the very same pain receptors that respond to actual heat. Chili pungency is not technically a taste; it is the sensation of burning, mediated by the same mechanism that would let you know that someone had set your tongue on fire."

The Scoville scale is used to measure the intensity of heat in peppers; it was developed by Wilbur Lincoln Scoville in 1912. Bell pepper is ranked as zero on the

Scoville scale; pure capsaicin is ranked at over 15 million SHU.

A jalapeno pepper ranges from 2500 to 8000 SHU, and a Scotch Bonnet pepper measures as high as 350,000. Ghost chilies, one of the hottest peppers, measure around 900,000 SHU.

Burning Sensation Equals Pain Relief

Capsaicin is able to help alleviate pain mainly by getting rid of what is known as substance P. This is a chemical component of all of the nerve cells that work to help transmit pain signals to the brain. The same substance is also what de-sensitizes the sensory receptors in the skin.

This is the reason why it is commonly added to cream that is used as a topical pain relieving medicine, as well as in patches, which can sometimes be ranked as 10 million SHU. Ironically, the very intense burning sensation is what provides the pain relief.

Capsaicin is most often used for relieving pain associated with shingles and HIV neuropathy, but it is also very helpful in relieving all types of joint pain including neck, back, and shoulder.

One research study examined a man who had persistent pain because of the wounds he received from a bomb explosion, and he was able to experience an 80 percent reduction in pain after using an 8% capsaicin patch.

A low concentration, 0.025%, topical capsaicin cream is helpful in relieving the pain caused by osteoarthritis. 80% of patients were able to experience a reduction in pain after only two weeks of four-times a day treatment.

It has also been found to help in reducing or eliminating the redness, itching, stinging and burning of skin due to moderate to severe psoriasis. A 2009 study examining a nasal spray that contained capsaicin found that it was able to significantly reduce allergy symptoms.

How is Capsaicin Used?

There are two main forms of capsaicin:

Capsaicin cream – This is common for most types of pain relief. Doctors will often suggest creams, ointments, films, sticks, gels, ointments, or lotions. These do not require prescriptions. This form will be thoroughly rubbed into your skin in the area where you are hurting and reapplied throughout the day. Make sure that you thoroughly wash your hands after you use the cream. Make sure the cream doesn't go near your mouth or eyes, or any other mucous membrane.

Capsaicin patches – This has higher amounts of capsaicin than the cream. This is often suggested by doctors for shingles pain and diabetic neuropathy. These can only be acquired from doctors. The doctor will numb the area and then apply the patch. This normally takes around two hours.

This patch has the ability to help relieve pain for up to three months. Avoid messing with the patch while it is on.

Side Effects

While capsaicin is fairly safe, the patches and creams can irritate the skin and cause some of the following:

- Pain
- Itching and burning
- Dryness
- Soreness
- Swelling and redness

This will often become worse in humid and hot weather, when bathing in warm water, and when sweating, but typically only lasts for a couple of days but can last for two to four weeks.

You will need to make sure you use sunscreen because capsaicin can make your skin more sensitive to heat and sun. Some people can be allergic to capsaicin. Contact your doctor if you experience trouble breathing, chest tightness, swelling in your throat, hives, and itching.

There are rare side effects from using the patch that can affect your heart, but these include a sudden increase or decrease in heart rate and blood pressure changes. Make sure your doctor knows your history of any heart problems, blood vessel problems, or if you suffer from high blood pressure.

Turmeric

Chances are you, have probably heard people rave over the health benefits of turmeric. There are loads of research that looked further into the vitamins and macronutrients in foods to phytochemicals and micronutrients.

The majority of the benefits of turmeric come from its anti-inflammatory and antioxidant potential and its ability to create homeostasis in the body. Because of this, people have started to turn towards eating healthful whole foods again, and turmeric's curcumin is the heaviest hitter when it comes to phytonutrients.

For example, curcumin has been found to be more effective than celecoxib to treat arthritis pain. Curcumin has antifungal, antioxidant, and antiviral properties. It also works to inhibit the function of molecules that cause inflammation because it contains COX-2 inhibitors. COX-2 is an enzyme that causes the formation of prostanoids, which is a fatty acid that causes an inflammatory reaction. This is also influenced by chronic inflammation caused by metabolic oxidation that the body goes through every day, local inflammation caused by minor injuries like cuts or scrapes, and post-surgical inflammation. Curcumin has no toxic effects to humans, so that means no prescription is needed.

Curcumin is able to reduce inflammation because it lowers histamine levels and stimulates the adrenal glands so that it will produce cortisone, which is your own natural painkiller. This can help to alleviate pain from:

- Ulcers – this only induces half the effect of OTC antacids, but it is a cheaper option. It also helps to work against *Helicobacter pylori*, which is the main cause of gastric ulcers.

- Gout

- Osteoarthritis – which is due to the mechanical wear and tear of the joints, such as the shoulder.

- Backache – this is caused by muscular pulls, strain, or sprains.

- Headache

- Kidney stones and gallstones – it works by thinning the bile and lowering stone formation or dissolving the already formed stone.

- Fibromyalgia

- Diverticulitis – this works by reducing the swelling of the colon pockets.

- Carpal tunnel syndrome

- Rheumatoid arthritis – this is caused by autoimmune dysfunction

There are also several other healing uses for turmeric.

- Mental decline – curcumin is able to bind with heavy metals like lead and cadmium, which reduces the toxicity of these heavy metals and protect the brain.

- Atherosclerosis – it is able to reduce the formation of blood clumps.

- Warts – it has proven to be active against the papillomavirus.

- Psoriasis – it helps to regulate inflammatory proteins that the immune system secretes; can be applied topically.

- Indigestion

- Viral infections

- Fungal infections – curcumin has at least 20 fungicidal compounds.

- Diabetes – it helps to increase insulin production and lowers blood sugar.

- Depression – it works similar to serotonin.

How Much to Take

Typically, you can take two tablespoons and mix it into the water to form a paste to use for topical applications, like arthritic joints or wounds. Internally, you can take a half to one and a half teaspoons of dried root powder each day. This would be 250 milligrams each day in the form of a supplement, or 400 to 600 milligrams of turmeric extract in a supplement for no more than three times a day for extreme pain.

It's a good idea to find a supplement that has black pepper in it as well, or you can add it in when cooking. Adding black pepper to your topical treatments for pain is extremely helpful.

If you plan on taking supplements for your pain, try to find those that are standardized to 95 percent curcuminoids, phospholipid-bound, and containing lecithin.

Adding turmeric to your regular diet is a great way to help prevent disease and pain. Ayurvedic medicine uses a lot of turmeric. Ayurvedic medicine is the traditional Indian healing practice. Here are some great ways to add turmeric to your diet:

- Use it for what it is, a spice, in main dishes like soups, beans, vegetables, rice, turkey, and chicken.

- Mix it into salad dressings, sautéed onions, eggs, bone broth, smoothies, potatoes, glazes, and marinades.

- Curry paste can be purchased, or you could make your own and mix it into soups or stir-fries.

- Add some onto cruciferous vegetables like kale, brussels sprouts, broccoli, cauliflower. The phenethyl isothiocyanates that the crucifers contain combine with curcumin to reduce your risk of prostate tumors.

- Adding in black pepper helps to improve the bioavailability of curcumin.

- Turmeric tea or golden milk is also a great option.

There are over 7000 studies that have found that turmeric can help beat all types of pain, including back, neck, and shoulder pains.

Ginger

Do you have ginger in your spice rack? Maybe you need to move it to your medicine cabinet. Besides the fact that it is a tasty spice, which is often used in holiday treats, ginger is able to diminish nausea and soothe upset stomachs, and studies have found that it can help ease inflammation and pain.

All through history, ginger has been a common treatment for digestive problems and nausea. Now science has found that it is also beneficial for those with chronic pain like arthritis.

In fact, a study at the University of Miami found that ginger extract could end up being a substitute for nonsteroidal anti-inflammatory drugs. Their study examined 247 patients and the effects of highly concentrated ginger extract to osteoarthritis of the knee. The ginger was able to reduce the stiffness and pain in the joints by 40% over the placebo.

During the six-week double-blind study, the participants were given either a highly concentrated ginger extract made from *Alpinia galangal* and *Zingiber officinale* or a placebo.

Beneficial Properties

Why is ginger so amazing? Ginger has antioxidant, anti-inflammatory, and anti-ulcer properties, and they have a small amount of analgesic property.

Research studies have found that the benefits of ginger come from several different compounds, which includes shogaols and gingerols. All of these compounds have anti-oxidant and anti-inflammatory properties. Besides being helpful for treating arthritis, ginger is also great for treating heart or digestive conditions and even cancer.

Its anti-inflammatory agents help get rid of pain and improve arthritis symptoms. Ginger's compounds work like COX-2 inhibitors, in the same way as traditional medications for psoriatic arthritis and rheumatoid arthritis.

The University of Georgia did another study built on previous work that identified ginger's success as an anti-inflammatory agent in rodents. A professor from the kinesiology department, Patrick O'Connor, led two studies that looked at how heat-treated and raw ginger affected muscle pain. The 74 participants consumed either heat-treated or raw ginger over an

11-day period and then took part in moderately tax arm exercises.

The effects were amazing. The ginger reduced the pain in both groups of participants by more than 25%, with both types of ginger providing nearly the exact same results. O'Connor said that this kind of exercise-induced pain is a very common pain across all activities. Ginger is able to help reduce this type of pain by reducing the inflammation in the muscle.

Osteoarthritis, which is a common cause of chronic shoulder, back, and neck pain, is one of the most common forms of arthritis and nearly 20 to 27 million people in the US suffer from it. This wear-and-tear condition tends to affect the larger, weight-bearing joints.

The majority of the studies on the anti-inflammatory and anti-oxidant properties of ginger have mainly been studied in rodents, but across everything, the results have shown a strong potential for human pain relief. There was one study that discovered that fresh ginger had good potential for anti-oxidant properties that were healing and protective when it came to cellular stress.

As far as its anti-inflammatory effects, studies have found that the different compounds found in ginger are able to help with pain in a variety of ways. One particular study found that ginger extract was able to reduce the elevated expression of TNF-a and NFkB in rats with liver cancer. Elevated levels of these compounds are typically linked to inflammatory diseases such as arthritis, diabetes, Crohn's, asthma, allergy, and cardiovascular disease.

Even though there aren't a lot of human research and trials, it does look as if ginger is able to help with pain specifically as it relates to inflammation.

Adding Ginger to Your Diet

Picking the best form of ginger is probably one of the biggest challenges to reaping its reward. You can get ginger in oils, powders, teas, tinctures, capsules, and foods made from the fresh or dried roots of the ginger plant.

Experts say that the best way to reap the benefits of ginger is to consume it in a 100 to 225 mg supplement. Make sure that you talk to your doctor first before you add this supplement to your diet. Ginger can interfere with blood-thinning medications such as warfarin. When picking out a supplement, try to find brands that use the words "super-critical extraction," because it provides you with the purest ginger and the best effect. It's best if you take your supplement along with food because too much ginger on an empty stomach can upset it.

While they smell great, foods such as ginger tea, gingerbread, and gingersnaps might not contain enough ginger to receive the needed benefits. Once your doctor says it's okay to try a ginger supplement, start out with 100 to 200 mg capsules, taking one a day for four to six weeks to see how strong dosage you need.

If you like to have that tangy zip of fresh ginger, I've got great news. Georgia State College & University in Milledgeville and the University of Georgia in Athens found that just a few added tablespoons of fresh ginger are able to ease exercise muscle pain.

Mix a few tablespoons into your food by grating the ginger into a stir-fry or over a salad. You can also grate some into a pot of hot water and let it steep for five minutes to make a soothing tea.

Before Using Ginger

While ginger is a lot safer to use than prescription strength painkillers, it can create problems with certain medications. Here are four things to remember before you start supplementing ginger.

1.   Check in with your doctor.

Before you start to add in a significant amount of ginger to your diet, speak with your doctor about any of the possible issues, which include drug interactions. This is extremely important for people who take Coumadin because ginger can reverse the effects of the drug.

2.   Pick the correct formulation

After you have spoken with your doctor, this probably is the most important part. As stated earlier, supplements are probably the best way to go. While many of the other options in this book work best when rub onto the skin in a tincture or cream form, ginger works best from the inside out. Follow the instructions from earlier to figure out the dosage you need. Keep in mind that 225 mg of ginger is almost equivalent to a bushel of fresh ginger, so that would be quite hard to eat in a single day.

3. Dose correctly.

Your doctor can also help you to pick the right dosage for you if you're not interested in playing the guessing game. Your doctor will start you out with 100 mg of ginger each day and test up to 200 mg for four to six weeks. You will have to keep track of any changes in your pain levels and your mobility.

4. Incorporate ginger into your life.

Whether you're supplementing with ginger or not, you can add more ginger into your daily life in many different forms. Keep some ginger root on hand and add to foods. Ginger freezes well, so keep some peeled ginger in your freezer and cut of one-inch squares and add to boiling water to create a tea.

Select, Prepare, and Store

When you buy ginger in the grocery store, it is likely ten months old. The skin is darker, and a little tough, and the inside is dark yellow. In some mature ginger, there can be a blue streak running through it. This ginger is Hawaiian blue ring ginger and is typically only available between December and April. This is a very pungent and juicy ginger.

Young ginger has a thinner skin that you won't have to peel before you use it. The flesh of the ginger is less fibrous and tough, which is the reason why it is the best ginger for creating that pile of pink ginger that comes along with sushi.

When you see a large knot of ginger, this is referred to as a hand. Try to find a firm and unwrinkled hand that doesn't have any signs of mold. If you are only looking for a small piece, it is okay to break off what you need. There are some Chinese medicine practitioners that believe that the best piece of ginger for medicinal use is a piece that is shaped like a person.

Whether you purchase a small piece or a large one that looks like a mini person, you can store ginger in the refrigerator packed in a loosely wrapped paper towel in a sealed plastic container. You can also freeze ginger in a plastic container. The best thing about freezing is that it can be grated more easily. Ginger can last for several weeks when stored in the fridge, and several months when frozen.

Make sure you peel the ginger before you store it. This can be done easily and safely with a spoon.

Devil's Claw

A lot of people who suffer from arthritis, as well as other types of back or joint pain, are turning to Devil's claw for help. Devil's claw is probably the most common home remedy for pain. But Devil's claw doesn't just help with pain. Much like turmeric, Devil's claw is a natural anti-inflammatory. Devil's claw is used like the South American cat's claw root to treat digestive problems and arthritis.

It tends to also be used along with bromelain to help relieve different types of joint pain, especially when it is caused by arthritis.

Devil's claw can provide many other health benefits other than pain relief. There is even one report that has studied its possibility of anticancer potential.

To fully understand what Devil's claw does, you need to understand what it is. Devil's claw is the *Harpogophytum procumbens* plant, which is a plant that is located in the Kalahari savanna of Southern Africa, Namibian steppes, and Madagascar.

Supplements of Devil's claw are typically made up of its dried roots. European and African folk and traditional medical practitioners have given attention to Devil's claw for more than 100 years to help with some pregnancy symptoms, relieve pain, reduce fever, and digestive ills.

It's believed that Devil's claw's benefits come from its content of iridoid glucosides, including harpagoside. These iridoids work as anti-inflammatories that are commonly found in plants and bind with glucose molecules. This is the reason why the compounds are known as iridoid glucosides. The European Scientific Cooperative on Phytotherapy says that Devil's claw contains at least 1% harpagoside.

Devil's claw also has phytosterols and bioflavonoids, which are plant-based antioxidants that have antispasmodic properties. These are helpful for treating digestive problems.

France even allowed marketing for Devil's claw claiming that it is "traditionally used for symptomatic relief of painful joint disorders." ESCOP has approved the use of Devil's claw for dyspepsia, loss of appetite, tendonitis, and painful arthritis.

In Greek, *Harpagophytum* translates to "hook plant." Growing originally and predominantly in Africa, the plant appears like it is covered with hooks. These hooks protect the fruit that grows on the plant, which allows it to be able to attach to the fur of animals to help spread its seeds.

There are several different uses for Devil's claw, which include reducing headache, back and chest pain, soothing heartburn, relieving the symptoms of gout, and boosting heart health.

Western medicine was introduced to the powers of Devil's claw root by South African farmer, G.H. Mehnert, who noticed how the natives use the plant. The first use of the plant in Europe was in 1953, where they used it for allergies, bladder, kidney, bile, liver, and arthritic complaints.

There was one study performed on Devil's claw where patients suffered from slight to moderate muscular tension, or slight muscular pain in the neck, back and shoulder. Using a double-blind, randomized basis, 31 participants were given doses of the extract of Devil's claw two times a day, and another 32 participants were given a placebo. The therapy lasted for four weeks. They achieved a highly significant clinical efficacy in cases of slight to moderate muscular pain.

Using Devil's Claw and Side Effects

Devil's claw can be used as a tea or in pill form. To get the benefits of Devil's claw, the plant's root is dried and packed into a tablet or capsule. It can also be used to make a liquid extract or an ointment to rub onto the skin. If you want to make a tea, you can brew four to five grams of the root in a cup of hot water. Drink this once a day for relief from muscle and joint pain.

If you want to take a supplement, try to find a product that contains extracts of Devil's claw with a standard of two to three percent iridoid glycosides. Make sure that the supplement comes from a safe company with a proven track record, and they list all ingredients and facts. Depending on the intensity of your pain, you can take 200 to 2500 mg each day. Start with 200 and increase the dosage until you receive relief from pain. Make sure you take a dosage for at least a week before increasing it.

There isn't much information as to the possible side effects. There are some sources that suggest that you shouldn't take it if you're breastfeeding or pregnant because they don't know what could happen.

WebMD says that people who have a peptic ulcer, gallstones, diabetes, low blood pressure, hypertension, or heart problems should steer clear from Devil's claw. There is a little bit of evidence that could suggest that it can affect these conditions. This means that if you suffer from one or more of these conditions, you should make sure to speak with health care provider and stay closely monitored.

There are some medications that might interact with Devil's claw. This includes medications that affect the liver because Devil's claw can slow down the liver's breakdown of the drugs. Warfarin is one such drug that could be affected by Devil's claw.

Other Benefits

1. Arthritis Relief

Curing osteoarthritis symptoms have been the most studied use of Devil's claw. A Japanese study performed in 2010 found that Devil's claw was able to reduce inflammation due to arthritis in mice.

Overall, Devil's claw is virtually accepted by the majority of doctors as a "supportive treatment for degenerative, painful rheumatism." Rheumatic diseases are marked by chronic inflammation and are typically located in the joint, fibrous, and muscle tissue pain.

When Devil's claw was tested on different rheumatic disorders, there was a significant reduction of pain in the back, knee, hip, shoulder, elbow, wrist, and hand. The same study also found that the patient's quality of life was improved. In fact, 60 % of participants ended up being able to reduce or quit using their pain medication.

Besides reducing pain, Devil's claw could possibly help prevent bone loss. The majority of tests have only been performed in labs on animals, but there are still lots of promising signs that the plant can prevent bone loss in inflammatory osteoporosis.

2. Weight Loss

The anti-inflammatory root could be able to help you lose weight. An Irish study discovered that Devil's claw was able to stop or slow down the production of ghrelin, which is the hunger hormone. By lowering hunger pangs, people who suffer from overeating issues could find that their appetites are lowered to average, which will aid in weight loss.

It could also end up helping to prevent weight-related atherosclerosis through the way that it is able to suppress inflammation.

3. Natural Painkiller

The pain benefits don't just work for arthritis pain. Even though they don't quite understand why, Devil's claw is able to reduce inflammation and the pain that it causes in several different conditions, including pain that is acute.

Some sources have also stated that Devil's claw is a great medication for sciatica. It's important to know, though, that there haven't been any studies performed on its effects on sciatica.

4. Fight's Chronic Inflammation

The most valuable part of Devil's claw is how it is able to lower inflammation throughout the body, which is one of the main causes of most diseases. Some of the most recent research has been able to find that Devil's claw is able to inhibit TBF-a, which is a cytokine that is a part of the regular inflammation response that happens throughout the body as it works to regulate your immune system.

This is a very important part of the body because whenever TNF-a is working harder than it should be, chronic inflammation will end up happening, which can then end up leading to several different types of diseases. The majority of studies aiming to prevent inflammatory diseases like IBD, psoriatic arthritis, psoriasis, and rheumatic diseases tries to determine how to inhibit TNF-a.

Cloves

When a person hears the word clove, they are often thinking about garlic cloves. Much like garlic, which we will talk about next, the health benefits of the herb clove dates back to over 2000 years. They are pretty amazing.

In tropical climates, cloves are typically harvested by hand, and it comes from the cute little unopened pink flower buds that grow on the evergreen clove tree. It looks similar to little pretzel sticks or even tiny nails.

Its hard exterior helps to protect the active elements in cloves, which is the light-yellow oil called eugenol, which is what contributes the majority of its health benefits and makes it a natural anti-inflammatory.

After it received a write up in the *New York Times*, cloves gained in popularity as a health item. The article stated that a common health benefit of using clove oil was as a safe and natural alternative of the more commonly used analgesics that contained benzocaine for toothaches.

A gel that was clove-based work just as well as benzocaine for treating patients who received needle stick on both sides of the gums five times over a ten-minute period as compared to people who received a placebo.

These findings were right on track with the use of eugenol extracts used in American dentistry and OTC mouthwashes, throat sprays, and toothpaste.

A study recently done by Miguel Hernandez University went straight to the biggest benefit of cloves. The researchers found that cloves were the top natural antioxidant spice that can and should be used in the food industry because of its natural high levels of phenolic compounds, as well as its antioxidant capacity.

Experts also consider cloves to be a nutrient-dense spice. Two ounces of cloves have 63 % of the daily value of manganese that humans need, along with vitamin C, dietary fiber, vitamin K, and omega-3 fatty acids.

Since cloves are so nutrient dense, cloves have been given the best score in the Oxygen Radical Absorption Capacity that was created by Tufts University for the USDA.

A single drop of clove essential oil can provide you with 400 times more antioxidants per unit volume than the magical goji berries. You can look at a 15-milliliter bottle of clove essential oil and compare it to the antioxidant power of 40 quarts of blueberries.

Clove is often used as an expectorant and used to treat an upset stomach. Clove oil is also great for bad bread, diarrhea, and hernia. Cloves can also be used to help with vomiting, nausea, and gas.

Clove is also often used on the skin to help ease pain and can be used for throat and mouth inflammation. When it comes to manufacturing, clove is often used in cigarettes, perfumes, cosmetics, soaps, and toothpaste.

Early research has found that applying a gel that contains ground cloves for five minutes before being struck by a needle is able to reduce the pain from the stick, similar to benzocaine.

Safety of Cloves

Used as a food additive, clove is safe for the majority of people to take by mouth. There isn't enough information about its safety when the clove is taken in a large medicinal amount.

It is perfectly safe to use cream or oil that contains clove when applied to the skin. However, repeated and frequent applications of clove oil on the gums or in the mouth can cause damage to the mucous membranes, skin, tooth pulp, and gums.

Children should not take clove oil by mouth. It can cause severe side effects like fluid imbalances, liver damage, and seizures. It should be safe to consume food containing cloves when pregnant or breastfeeding. Medicinal amounts of clove have not been studied, so if you are pregnant or breastfeeding, stay safe, and avoid medicinal doses.

Some anticoagulant drugs can be affected by cloves. Cloves can slow down clotting, so be careful.

Using Cloves

Cloves are typically taken in supplement form. The most common form of cloves is the essential oil. You can also add cloves to recipes to add flavor and health benefits.

When using clove oil, make sure that you dilute the oil in a carrier oil. Full strength could end up irritating your skin.

Garlic

There is a theoretical benefit of garlic, and that is arthritis and pain relief when consumed orally. There are also several other ways that you can take garlic. Garlic can be eaten cooked or raw. You can also find it in dried or powdered form, as well as in tablets or capsules. You can also find garlic in liquid extracts and in oils. It's important that you speak with your doctor before you start to take a garlic supplement for a natural pain remedy.

Garlic contains anti-inflammatory and antioxidant properties that are able to help ease the pain from arthritis and other types of joint pain. There was a study published in the *Soviet Archives of Internal Medicine* in 1999 that stated that garlic taken twice a day for four to six weeks was able to work just as well for rheumatoid arthritis as conventional therapy. However, not every single study on the use of garlic for pain provides positive results. For example, if you take garlic for leg pain during walking that is caused by poor circulation due to peripheral arterial disease, you probably won't reap any benefits.

Another great attribute of garlic is that it is able to increase the potency of nonsteroidal anti-inflammatory drugs that you take to help with pain. This means that you will receive an even greater relief from pain. However, if you want to try this, make sure that you talk to your doctor first. Garlic is also able to add to the effects of other drugs. For example, garlic is also able to magnify the effects of blood-thinning drugs such as warfarin and aspirin. Garlic oil is also able to decrease how fast the liver is able to break down certain types of medications. This can end up increasing the medications effects and side effects. Some examples include chlorzoxazone, acetaminophen, and theophylline, and even drugs that are used for anesthesia during surgery such as isoflurane and halothane.

The selenium content of garlic is what makes it helpful for managing arthritis pain or even preventing arthritis. Garlic contains novel sulfur compounds, one such compound is called thiacremonone. This is able to help inhibit your body's inflammatory responses, which means it is a useful agent when it comes to treating inflammatory and arthritic diseases.

The antioxidant content of garlic is also able to reduce

inflammation, and thus it will help to manage pain. Antioxidant nutrients are able to help reduce the inflammatory symptoms that come along with inflammatory joint diseases.

Amazing Facts

The following facts came from the University of Maryland Medical Center, *Journal of Immunology Research*, and *Journal of Immunology*.

- All plants that come from the genus Allium are known for producing organic sulfur compounds, which contain interesting pharmacological and biological properties. Garlic is among this group, *Allium sativum*, which is the most widely used.

- When they are isolated and extracted, these compounds exhibit a large spectrum of healthful effects that fight against microbial infections, which are also used to help protect against heart disease.

- Currently, they are looking at how garlic can help to boost the immune system, and even fight cancer.

- One of garlic's potent sulfur-based compounds is allicin, which is responsible for the smell of garlic but is probably also the reason for its antibacterial properties.

Benefits

People will often refer to garlic as the "stinking rose," but it does seem to have a full bouquet of benefits. But it also matters how you prepare it. Research has found that if you heat garlic too soon, it will interfere with the health benefits that come from allicin.

This means that if you have crushed, minced, or chopped garlic, allow it to sit for five to ten minutes before you cook it. If you can't wait, and you go ahead and throw it into some hot oil or boiling water, all you are doing is deactivating its beneficial enzyme. Patience is most definitely a virtue when you are preparing this golden nugget.

Another great thing about garlic is that it is cheap. A head of garlic isn't that expensive, and you can even sometimes find them in groups of three. You can also buy an expensive jar of pre-chopped garlic, which equals several cloves. This means that it is a cheap option for pain relief.

To take your garlic, you have several options. One way to consume your garlic is to eat a clove every morning. Some people will finely chop or grate it, allow it to rest for five to ten minutes, and then mix it into water and drink it. You can also incorporate more garlic into your cooking. It's best to aim for two to three cloves of fresh garlic every day to help treat your shoulder, neck, or back pain. Most websites will recommend you consume them first thing in the morning, but you can also mix them into your foods so that it's not so strong. Just make sure you let it rest before you cook it.

Another way to get pain relief from garlic is through a garlic oil rub. This works as a topical analgesic. Place ten whole cloves of garlic in two ounces of sesame or coconut oil. Allow the oil to heat and cook the garlic until they turn brown. Strain the garlic cloves out of the oil and store the oil in a small glass jar. Make sure you use the oil within the next few days.

If you want to take a supplement, you can find supplements that range from 150 mg to 2400 mg. You will have to test to see which strength works best for your pain level.

Safety

It appears that garlic is safe for the majority of adults, but it is best if you talk to your doctor before taking a supplement, especially if you are currently on any medicine or have a health condition. Garlic can even interfere with the effectiveness of the drug saquinavir, an HIV drug. Some possible side effects could include allergic reactions, an upset stomach, body and breath odor, and heartburn. If you already have a bleeding disorder, garlic may make it worse because of the blood-thinning properties. If you have planned surgery or dental work, you need to use garlic with caution.

Marjoram

When people use marjoram for pain, they use its essential oil. Sweet marjoram oil is created from the steam distillation of the tops of the plant, and it is a cousin of oregano. The resulting yellow-green essential oil has a camphoraceous, woody, spicy, and warm scent that will remind you of cardamom and nutmeg.

Meanwhile, you also have Spanish marjoram oil, which is a different essential oil that comes from marjoram plants, and it has a red-orange hue. This marjoram was originally native to the Mediterranean areas and North America, today it is widely grown for large-scale commercial use of its oil in Spain, Tunisia, Germany, France, Egypt, and, recently, the United States.

According to folklore, the Egyptians would dedicate the marjoram plant to Osiris, the god of the underworld. They used it to produce love potions, unguents, and medicines. The Romans and Greeks consider this herb to be an herb of happiness and they offered it to the goddess of beauty, love, and fertility, Aphrodite.

In the culinary world, sweet marjoram is an excellent way to add flavor to salads, soups, and other delicious dishes.

Marjoram tea is also popular among women to help promote a better flow of breast milk and ease menopausal symptoms. Sweet marjoram oil will also provide you with positive effects when used in:

- Topical applications as lotion, salve, or cream.

- Massage therapy when it is mixed in with a mild carrier oil or added to bath water.

- Vapor therapy through vaporizers and burners,

When it is used as an inhalant or with aromatherapy, sweet marjoram oil works great for people with insomnia and can't settle down for bed.

Composition

The main chemical make-up of sweet marjoram oil is y-terpineol, terpinene-4-ol, linalyl acetate, cissabinene hydrate, Linalool, terpinolene, p-cymene, y-terpinene, a-terpinene, and sabinene. The oil mixes perfectly with tea tree, eucalyptus, bergamot, chamomile, cedarwood, cypress, and lavender.

How it Works

There are lots of different health benefits that you can get from marjoram, but since we are focusing on pain, here is how it helps different types of pain:

- Analgesic – it helps to alleviate pain related to headache, toothache, inflammation, fevers, and colds.

- Emmenagogue – it helps to regulate painful and irregular menstrual periods.

Safety and Side Effects

If used appropriately, sweet marjoram is perfectly safe. However, it is best if you don't use it, or pretty much any essential oil, if you have an existing condition, or if you are breastfeeding or pregnant. Since it does have emmenagogue properties, which stimulates blood flow, you should never use sweet marjoram oil during pregnancy.

Sweet marjoram oil can also cause allergic reactions or hypersensitivity, so make sure you perform a patch test on a small area of skin to see how you could react to it when used topically. If you mix it with a mild carrier oil, it will help lessen its sensitizing effect.

How to Use

There are several different ways to use marjoram to relieve pain. The essential oil makes it extremely easy as well because you can add some to baths or massages for soothing effects. For a more specific pain like neck, back, or shoulder, dilute some marjoram oil into a cream. Rub the cream onto the painful area, and you will experience some relief.

Parsley

You are probably familiar with parsley as a fresh herb or dried spice, but it has also been proven to be amazing for your health. Even if you only eat parsley in a small amount, there are loads of health benefits because it is full of beneficial nutrients, antioxidants, and essential oil, so much that it is often referred to as a superfood.

It is derived from the Petroselinum plant. Parsley and its oil have been used as a natural anti-inflammatory, antiseptic, diuretic, and detox remedy for centuries. Today, many research studies have started to back up health claims that everybody else has believed for years.

In the *Journal of Traditional Chinese Medicine*, a study was published in 2013 that said parsley has been used to help treat various dermal diseases, diabetes, urinary disease, cardiac disease, hypertension, and gastrointestinal disorder.

The amazing benefits of parsley come from its active ingredient, which includes nutrients such as vitamins

A, K, and C, essential oils such as apiol and myristicin, antioxidant flavonoids, and phenolic compounds.

This means that parsley is an all-natural and safe plant that you can add to your diet so that you can reap its digestion, antifungal, antibacterial, antidiabetic, brain protector, heart protector, and radical scavenger benefits.

Even though there is still more formal research needed, there is already strong evidence associated with parsley's ability to fight the following disorders and symptoms:

- Skin problems

- Poor immunity

- Constipation

- Acid reflux

- Gas

- Edema or bloating

- Arthritis

- Bad breath

- Kidney stones

- Digestive problems

- Bladder infection

- Anemia

- Oxidative stress or free radical damage

- Inflammation

- Pain relief

Parsley has been used for decades to help relieve pain associated with arthritis and other joint diseases. It is packed full of vitamin K, magnesium, and calcium, which all help to reduce the inflammation that causes pain.

Consuming parsley also leads to faster excretion of uric acid. This will end up leading to less joint stiffness and swelling that is associated with uric acid. It is also a great cure for osteoarthritis because it promotes bone health. It contains folate and calcium, which helps to protect the bone from wearing down.

Consuming Parsley

It is believed that drinking parsley tea throughout the day will help improve your joint range of motion. Here is a great recipe for parsley tea:

- Boil eight ounces of water.

- Rinse off a quarter cup of fresh parsley leaves in cool water.

- Pat them dry and roughly chop them. You can also leave them whole, but chopping will release some of the oil, which makes the tea stronger.

- Add the leaves to a cup and cover with the boiling water.

- Steep for ten minutes and then strain out the leaves.

- Sweeten with a bit of honey if needed, and enjoy.

You should try to drink half a cup of tea before breakfast and then another half before dinner. If you have a flare up of pain, you can drink another half cup.

Any unused tea can be refrigerated for later use. This tea is a great way to receive several different minerals and vitamins.

You don't just have to consume parsley in tea form. It is a delicious herb to add to different types of foods. There are also several different varieties of parsley out there. Italian flat leaf is fragrant, while curly parsley is a little more bitter. There are several other types as well, way too many to list. Parsley is a very versatile herb to cook.

Italian flat leaf parsley is great for salads and sauces. Curly leaf parsley is great for seasonings on chicken and beef.

Rosemary

A popular essential oil that is being used today is extracted from the *Rosmarinus officinalis* plant. This plant is very well known throughout the Mediterranean for its herbal and culinary benefits. It has been used for many health purposes.

Rosemary is related to mint but looks a lot like lavender. Its leaves look like flat pine needles that have been brushed with silver. It has a woodsy, citrusy fragrance that has become popular in many apothecaries, gardens, and kitchens all over the world. It got its name from the Latin words "ros" meaning dew and "marinus" meaning sea or simply "dew of the sea."

An old legend states that the Virgin Mary placed her blue wrap over a rosemary bush while she took a rest. The white flowers then turned blue. The bush then became known as the "Rose of Mary."

Rosemary is sacred to the Romans, Greeks, Hebrews, and Egyptians. It was used as protection against plagues and to scare off evil spirits. Rosemary essential oil is clear with a refreshing herbal smell. It can be a bit watery. Essential oils are made from the fresh flowers by using steam. It will yield one to two percent.

Paracelsus, a German-Swiss physician, loved its health benefits. During the 1500s he helped people understand the benefits of herbal medicine. He loved rosemary oil due to its ability to strengthen the whole body. It could help heal organs such as the brain, heart, and liver.

Uses

Rosemary can be used as salad dressings along with thousands of other uses. It is very hardy and will grow very easy either inside or out. Add a whole sprig to soups for a one of a kind flavor. High-quality rosemary oil has expectorant, antioxidant, anti-inflammatory, anti-infection, antifungal, anticatarrhal, anticancer, antibacterial, and analgesic properties.

Here is a list of some health problems that rosemary oil can help you with:

- Clarity – Place a few drops in your hands, rub

them together to warm up the oil. Cup your hands over your nose and mouth for about one minute.

- Cough – Massage a couple drops over the throat and chest every couple of hours.

- Headaches – Place a few drops in your hands. Cup your hands over your nose and mouth for a minute. You could also apply a few drops topically to the part of your head that hurts.

- Memory and Learning – Diffuse the oils in the rooms you are occupying. Take a few whiffs straight from the bottle. Rub some on your temples. Apply to your toes every day.

- Vaginal Infections – Massage a few drops in and around the vaginal area. Test the area for sensitivity before you place it inside the vagina.

Rosemary teas and oils can be added to lotions and shampoos. By using the oil daily, it can help to stimulate the hair follicles. This will help with growing long, strong, and luscious hair. You could also massage the oil into your scalp to remove dandruff and nourish it.

You can also use rosemary oil on pets to help with hair growth. It will help their coats become shiny. It also helps to fight fungal infections in their ears.

Rosemary oil is a natural disinfectant and can be used as a mouthwash to help prevent bad breath. By getting rid of the bacteria in the mouth, it can prevent cavities, the build-up of plaque, and other dental problems. Rosemary has a mesmerizing aroma that makes it a wonderful inhalant.

Rosemary oil can be put into cosmetics, fresheners, bath oils, perfumes, and candles. It will give your mind and energy boost when inhaled. When diluted 50/50, you can apply rosemary oil to wrists and ankles, vitaflex and chakra points, inhaled, diffuse, or as a supplement.

Benefits

Rosemary oil has been studied and used since ancient times for many health benefits. It is still used today for the same purposes. These include the following:

- Indigestion – Rosemary oil can be used to relieve bloating, constipation, stomach cramps, and flatulence. It can be helpful to stimulate appetite. Researchers show that it can detoxify the liver. It can regulate how the liver creates and releases bile. This is the main part of our digestive process.

- Stress Relief – Rosemary can decrease the level of cortisol. This is the hormone the body releases in the salivary gland during the flight-or-fight process. One study shows that inhaling lavender and rosemary oils for about five minutes can reduce cortisol levels significantly. This decreases the dangers of chronic stress.

- Pain Relief – Rosemary oil has been widely known for its pain-relieving properties. It is used to treat arthritis, muscle pain, and headaches. Massage some oil onto the affected area. You could add it to hot bath water to help treat rheumatism. Its anti-inflammatory properties surely help to relieve pain from joint aches and sprains.

- Boost the Immune System – Studies show that inhaling the essential oil while massaging it into the affected area can increase free radical's scavenging activities. Antioxidants are needed to fight disease and infection. By inhaling or using rosemary oil regularly, it can give your immunity a boost to help you fight off diseases caused by free radicals.

- Respiratory problems – Inhaling rosemary oil can relieve and treat respiratory problems like the flu, sore throat, colds, allergies, and throat congestion. Because of its antiseptic properties, rosemary oil can be used to fight respiratory infections. Due to its antispasmodic properties, it can help treat bronchial asthma with specific treatment programs.

Rosemary oil does great things for anxiety. Using sachets that contain rosemary and lavender essential oils can reduce anxiety caused by taking tests.

Using rosemary can help brain health. Rosemary can help improve the moods of healthy adults. A study done over a month's time using aromatherapy that included orange, lavender, lemon, and rosemary oils increased the cognitive functions of Alzheimer's patients.

Making Infused Oil

Rosemary essential oil is so versatile that it's so easy to use in aromatherapy with many different aromas. It can blend well with peppermint, chamomile, lemongrass, citronella, thyme, basil, sage, clary, frankincense, and lavender.

It is easy to make your own rosemary oil by putting a couple sprigs of totally dry rosemary into a glass jar. Fill the jar with olive oil. Put the lid on the jar and give it a slight shake. Store the jar in a dark, warm place for two weeks. Remove the rosemary sprigs. Keep the oil stored in the glass jar. For a fragrant bath, add ¼ cup to a tub of hot water. Blend with some balsamic vinegar for a tasty salad dressing.

How it Works

To help relieve congestion in the respiratory tract, pain, mental fatigue, and help blood circulation, use rosemary oil in vaporizers, burners, in a relaxing bath, or just massage it into the affected areas. To use as a hair and skin care agent, use blended oils in shampoos, conditioners, lotions, or creams. You only need to add about three drops of essential oil to a bath.

Safe?

Rosemary oil is an effective and safe oil that is good for a variety of purposes and uses. Before putting it directly onto your skin, dilute it with a carrier oil so it won't cause skin sensitivity. Always do a patch test first.

Breastfeeding or pregnant women should not use rosemary essential oils during pregnancy or while breastfeeding. Always talk to your doctor before giving rosemary oil to children. Never self-treat any chronic disease like Alzheimer's or depression with rosemary oil. This could cause serious problems if you haven't consulted your doctor first.

Side Effects

Sometimes rosemary might cause an allergic reaction. As said above, always talk to your doctor for proper usage. Due to the fact that it is volatile in nature, it could cause spasms and vomiting. Never ingest the essential oil. Again, pregnant women should never use rosemary essential oil as it can cause the miscarriage of an unborn child.

Thyme

For many years thyme has been used in many culinary dishes. It used to be used as a medicine by early Europeans. It was used to treat many different health problems.

Many people use thyme in puns, but nobody really knows where it originated. It is thought to have come from the ancient Greek word "thumus" that means courage. Other people think it came from the Egyptian word "tham" that means courage. Each one of these interpretations shows the main qualities of the herb.

Thyme is a short shrub that originates from the southern part of Europe. It has the smallest leaves of any shrub in a garden. Even though it is small in size, it has always symbolized bravery and strength for thousands of years in many cultures.

From the time of the ancient Greeks, this fragrant herb has been utilized to help overcome adversity and fear. Thyme has been used to help improve courage, overcome shyness, and alleviate depression. People who lived during the Renaissance used to put thyme under their pillow to ward off nightmares. It was also put into coffins to help loved ones enter into the afterlife in Europe.

Cough

Thyme isn't used as a medicine much anymore, but it has several medicinal properties. Other than putting it in your favorite foods, thyme can be used to help with congestion and coughing. Thyme can break up phlegm and will clear the head and chest. For thousands of years, it has been used to relieve the symptoms of influenza and colds. Dioscorides would drink thyme mixed with vinegar and salt to help get rid of phlegm by sending it through the bowels.

Thyme's drying effects make it great for colds and other conditions that cause the lungs to become congested by mucus. Thyme can be used to help control coughing spasms and can be used as an antitussive especially when battling whooping cough.

Scientists have started validating thyme's use in helping cure bronchitis. In a double-blind study, researchers saw that patients who are given dried extracts of thyme mixed with evening primrose had quicker a healing time than patients that were given a placebo.

In another study, researchers found that an extract of thyme mixed with ivy leaves controlled their patient's cough two days faster than patients who took a placebo. This combination is safe for children between the ages of two and 17.

Thyme can be used to help with the symptoms of upper-respiratory infections, whooping cough, and bronchitis. Thyme is one of the ten herbs found in the cough drop Ricola.

Purification

There are several cultures that practice the burning of dried thyme to purify their homes and temples. The fragrance has been described as earthy, bitter, but altogether pleasant.

It was thought that thyme can prevent evil spirits from entering the home or a person. One Roman doctor thought thyme could send away any venomous creatures.

Infection

Thyme contains chemicals called phytochemicals that help the body fight infections. Thyme can kill yeast, fungal, and bacterial infections. It can also kill parasites like roundworm and hookworm. Some herbalists will use thyme and other herbs in a vaginal suppository to help with Group B Streptococcus during the last stages of pregnancy.

Thyme belongs to the mint family and is rich in essential oils. This gives the plant its powerful scent and medicinal powers.

Ancient Sumerians used thyme like an antiseptic. Egyptians mummified their dead using thyme. Roman emperors would chew thyme after a meal thinking it would prevent them from being poisoned. During the Victorian
Age, nurses would disinfect bandages by washing them in thyme water.

Thyme's ability to fight microbes is the main reason it is used to preserve food and can be used to fight many different types of bacterial infections. You can use it as a wash for minor mouth infections, inflamed gums, or sore gums. Making a gargle with honey that has been infused with thyme can help soothe a sore throat. Listerine has used thyme oil in its mouthwash since 1879 to help kill germs that cause bad breath.

Thyme can inhibit the properties that cause bacterial cells to become resistant to antibiotics. There are an estimated two million people who get antibiotic-resistant infections every year in the United States. These infections could result in over 23,000 deaths. Thyme along with other herbs that have the same properties might be that ray of hope to help with the threat of antibiotic-resistant bacteria.

Digestion

Just like most herbs, thyme tastes amazing but also helps with digestion. It can be eaten in meals to support a healthy digestive system. If needed, it can be taken in bigger amounts to help with flatulence, belching, and bloating. It can help to calm digestive spasms to help with irritable bowel syndrome or diarrhea.

Pain

Most people don't think that a common herb would have the ability to help relieve pain, but thyme has the ability to cure headaches and sciatica. Some people believe that thyme is as good as clove for an oral anesthetic. Thyme oil was used during World War I to help treat wounds.

Researchers continue to uphold thyme's reputation as a pain reliever. One study found that essential oil made from thyme could relieve menstrual cramps just as well as ibuprofen. It actually works better with time. Women in the ibuprofen group said their cramps weren't relieved as well during the second month. The thyme group said the oil gave more pain relief during the second month.

Thyme essential oil can be rubbed on painful joints. Thyme can be used for gout, and normal everyday aches and pains.

Uses

Thyme is a very popular culinary herb since it goes well with almost everything. It can be a bit spicy and bitter, so take it easy. Thyme gives a pleasing flavor and helps with digestion.

You can throw the entire sprig of thyme into whatever you are cooking. Just remember to remove all the stems before serving the dish. You can tie the thyme with some kitchen twine to help you remove the stems faster.

Thyme tea is a great choice when choosing a medicinal tea. Think about this recipe from Hippocrates: Boil two cups of water with three tablespoons of thyme. Cover the pot and let it steep for ten minutes. Drink two glasses each day to help with bronchitis.

Thyme can be prepared as a tea or a tincture which is an alcohol extract. It can also be infused with honey, vinegar, or oil.

You can find thyme essential oil in either white or red. Red is a lot stronger and will cost more. It can also cause skin irritation. The white oil has been refined. You should use both sparingly but never during pregnancy. To use it topically, dilute it with carrier oil like almond or coconut oil. Do not take thyme essential oil internally if you are not working with a practitioner who is qualified.

The best way to use essential oils is by using a diffuser. Take a whiff when you are in need of some courage.

Here are some dosage suggestions:

Thyme tea: two to six grams of dried tea to one cup boiling water each day.

Thyme Extract: dried thyme in a one to five ratio with 35 % alcohol. Take two to four milliliters three times each day.

Thyme Essential Oil: Dilutions of 1 % or fewer. Place one drop of essential oil to 100 drops of carrier oil.

Special Considerations

Thyme is very safe when used in small quantities.

Pregnant or nursing women shouldn't use thyme or thyme essential oil. If taken in large dosages, thyme can stimulate menstrual flow or uterine contractions.

Choose thyme due to its chemotype and use it only when diluted and in small amounts. Find an aromatherapist who has been trained on how to use essential oils internally. This will ensure that you take the right amount of this very potent extraction.

Allergic reactions are very rarely reported with thyme usage.

To Sum it up

Thyme is native to the sunny Mediterranean rocky soils. Thyme gives aromatic and powerful medicines in a very small package. Thyme can be eaten regularly in many meals. It can be added to beef dishes, salad dressings, and stews. You can drink tea made from thyme. It can also be made into a tincture. Thyme is great in helping with poor digestion. It also helps with influenza or colds. Research is being done to see how effective thyme can be against antibiotic-resistant bacterial infections.

Conclusion

Thank you for making it through to the end of *Physical Pain Herbal Medicine*, we hope it was informative and was able to provide you with all of the tools you need to achieve your goals whatever they may be.

The next step is to start trying some of these herbal remedies for your pain. Start with one or two and see what works best for you. Make sure that you follow recommended doses; otherwise, you may not get any relief. It's also a good idea to talk to your doctor first to make sure that the source of your pain isn't something major.

Finally, if you found this book useful in any way, a review on Amazon is always appreciated!

Description

Are you tired of dealing with your back, neck, or shoulder pain?

If you answered yes, then you need this book. The power of herbal medicine has been around for centuries, and it's still powerful today.

Prescription medicines and over-the-counter pain killers come with a lot of side effects, and possible addictions. Herbal medicines are a healthier option.

This book has ten herbal remedies that can help reduce pain and inflammation. You will learn about:

- Capsaicin

- Turmeric

- Ginger

- Devil's claw

- Cloves

- Garlic

- Marjoram

- Parsley

- Rosemary

- Thyme

Herbal remedies are a safe and great way to treat ailments without the side effects of Eastern medicine. Get this book today and say goodbye to your pain.

www.ingramcontent.com/pod-product-compliance
Lightning Source LLC
Chambersburg PA
CBHW070032260726

48658CB00002B/604